WALKING ALONG THE EDGE

Alden Sproull

WALKING ALONG THE EDGE

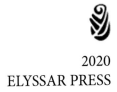

2020
ELYSSAR PRESS

Printed in the United States of America

First Printing, 2020

ISBN 978-1-733-4529-2-2

Elyssar Press
175 Bellevue Ave
Redlands, CA 92373

www.ElyssarPress.com

Cover Illustration Photo by Alden Sproull
Cover design by Stephanie Aoun @ 5D Studios
Book design and production by Stephanie Aoun @ 5D Studios
Editing by Allie Rigby @ Sunlight Editing Services

TABLE OF CONTENTS

Celebrating the Written Word!

Scratching Lines

Something Greater

THE EDGE!

You are vulnerable,
disease comes with its
cutting edge diagnosis, you,
have a serious illness.

Welcome the new faces,
agreeing to walk together
strengthens our ability to
be awake in each step.

The edge shared together
cuts both ways, hope being
shattered, then rebuilt
over and over again.

Hanging together teaches,
darkness is not the enemy.
It pushes us into the unknown,
then nudges us forward.

Here we see splashes of
light empowering us to let
go and embrace the
remaining gifts.

Edge living is full of pain, grief,
happiness, laughter and joy. Shared
love on the journey gives us
a new understanding of hope.

Truth comes to us through
honest connection with each other,
good or
bad.

Truth, often hard,
guides us to redefine
love, separation
and togetherness.

Coming to this intersection
for many is all
that has carried them
into the next day.

PREFACE

I wish to thank the patients from over the years, who have encouraged me to write these poems, and also to have them published so others could benefit from our shared journeys.

I wish to thank my wife, Victoria, for again having to look at the back of my head for hours on end as she did when writing my dissertation. She was open to read and react to what I was trying to convey. She has been a continuous support even when I couldn't recognize it.

Also, I am thankful for many of the staff nurses and physicians who supported me along the journey. They were the ones who initially gave me the referrals which started these walks.

I am grateful to Katia Hage, publisher at Elyssar Press, for her positive input along the way and challenging my doubts, would the collection ever come to completion.

I would also like to acknowledge Allie Rigby, the editor, for her work on this manuscript. Her insights and direction regarding suggested changes, her creativity influencing the design, and the poems'order have made the result a better collection. Thank you to each one who has aided in bringing this book of poetry to completion.

AUTHOR'S NOTES

Guidance for Reflecting with Poetry:

1. What attracts you to the poem you have before you?
2. Does anything in the poem trouble you?
3. What are you personally hearing in the poem?
4. What is the poem inviting you to become?
5. What would happen if you took the invitation seriously?

What words connect us to our feelings?

Give yourself time to feel the poem.

What feelings does this poem awaken in you?

What images in the poem break through the mind's rational surface to reveal emotions you may have ignored or suppressed?

Free associate with the lines of the poem. Do you feel sadness, relief, mystery, loneliness, warmth, respect, beauty, love?

Write whatever comes up for you.

Write freely.

What images arise that are connected with those feelings?

I apologize to these process pieces' originators for I do not recall where I picked them up.

Several poems came from writing with patients, any additional errors or misjudgments are mine.

INTRODUCTION

The definition of the word edge speaks to the life experience that formed the book's poetry.

Edge, according to Webster:
> the cutting side of a blade,
> the sharpness of a blade,
> penetrating power,
> keenness,
> a noticeably harsh quality,
> a point near the beginning and the end.

I chose to walk alongside many people who were struggling with serious illnesses. I discovered choosing this path meant I needed to accept that I didn't have more than an academic understanding of illness. I would need to be taught by those who were in the battle with being ill every day of their lives. For me, this meant walking the edge with them often between life and death.

What stands out today is the reality of accompaniment as I walked with them and their energy given to walk beside me. This worked well toward life and ministry shared together in some of the most challenging times of their lives.

Some have said to me, "You walk in where angels fear to tread."
I simply had faith believing a joint journey together will work, and I was always willing to give it a good try.

The years of the journey have been exciting, challenging, disturbing, troubling, and life-changing. The price regarding what I was asked to let go of and the gifts given in return have been greater blessings than money could ever buy.

The poems in this book are my attempts to capture what it meant to walk the edges in people's lives. Many of these poems have been shared with families, and some have found them clear pictures of their felt experience during their loved one's process.

These poems have been one of the treasured ways for me to continue the work over many years.

Webster's guidance fits well into what I felt on many days setting, listening, walking, holding, praying, celebrating, and grieving. The edge propelled me into the uncertain paths of life. We often were called upon to wrestle with the questions, Why am I here? Why is this happening to me?
After what I have been through, how can this be happening to me? How will my family cope?

One of the requirements upon entering this journey is the importance of a good listening ear. Listening is a sacred act, which lifts the spirit of the one speaking. Just to be heard is often what is necessary at the moment. I learned holding a hand spoke deeply to their lives more so than a lot of words. The held hand kept them steady in the current storms going on in their lives.

My actions conveyed that I deeply cared for them and couldn't walk away, no matter what was going on in their lives. This attitude provided the bridge to the next phase of our lives together, wherever it may have led.

As you walk through these poems, you will experience the cutting edge in your own life, pointing to your confusion, asking what this means for me? Those served would give you this guidance, take time for reflection, let insights go deeper, and trust the process. Who knows what you will discover?

ONE

CELEBRATING THE WRITTEN WORD

At the core of my work, there is a pure joy of writing. Writing is medicinal and is a beautiful "solution" to all the pain of existence which my poetry dives into.

CELEBRATING THE WRITTEN WORD!

Once written, they come alive,
breathing into the fiber of those
who wish to encounter them,
shifting the way one sees.

Thoughts come, move quickly,
stimulated by an intensity,
clashing words together in
our brains.

Submitting themselves to
a form, where permitted, to
enter the page as words, taking
on a clarity never known before.

The love of words
on a page, accepting
some order of design,
lifts my spirit into joy!

THE STIRRINGS

Hunger for a different life
stirs in our breast,
hoping for it to spring
forth.

Much like winter, our
inner workings are brought
to a gradual halt,
longing for the Celtic feast

of Imbolc, a time acknowledging
the stir of the earth, bringing forth,
new life, with a thriving hope.

Feel it coming…….
Are you open for its creative energy?

A PITCHER!

Spinning the wheel,
the potter discovers the
clay's intent. The hands working
the clay assist in its unfolding.

Agreement comes between clay
and potter,
a pitcher is formed,
handles added.

The pitcher cries
for water to carry,
just like a person
cries for work
that is real!

SHARED LIMITS

Pushing for a higher ideal_____
blocking my acceptance of
obvious limits, discovering they
are not shared well!

Acceptance of limits
usually brings a personal sense of
failure, unhappy with this,
I am.

Reminded of insurmountable feelings,
self-doubt emerges. Are these
shared limits, spiritual practice
toward deepening love and intimacy?
I wonder!

DROPPING THE STORY

Busy lives frustrate
our inner stories,
which long to be heard.
Stories once expressed,
with a grand acceptance,
shifting content toward
hopefulness, intense stories
need freedom to breathe, high
pitched emotions, vented, letting go
of what feeds the pain.
Left behind, they dictate how we feel,
what we see and how we respond.

GUITAR LADY...

She was playing the
guitar as I entered
the fountain area
this evening.

Turning quickly away,
not wanting to surprise her,
I move gently to a nearby
ledge to listen.

I know the longing of a soft
touch and a warm heart,
enfolded in her relationship
with the guitar and the music.

The music expresses itself
in a communion of hope and
healing. It challenges me as I am
surrounded by the duties of life.

She calls my desire to learn,
risk relationship with creativity.
She welcomes me to the edge
pushes me over, to fly.

HARD WORK TOWARD HEARING

Clutter and noise fill
so much of our lives, it seems
by choice, we distance ourselves
from the still small voice.

Choice fills our ears with noise
which must be dug out by the Spirit.
What are the (necessary) walls we build
keeping the Divine at a distance?

When our heart aches to be near,
held and welcomed. Maybe not as
grounded as we think,
our heart calls forth this prayer.

"Do with me as you wish."

RUNNING WHICH WAY?

I find myself at an intersection
of life, hesitating, it calls forth
some decision from me,
"Which way will I go?"

Will I find guidance, as I initially face
my deepest fears, intense anxieties?
What is there to uncover,
where to place my next steps?

I long to connect to a deeper
flow. Acknowledging my ache
for something more, gives me
greater assurance.

Afraid of needing others, to rouse
me awake, to push me over the edge
toward discovery,
fIlled now with wonder.

CAUGHT!

Caught in the cage of
discouragement,
breaking troubles, filled with the
emotions of betrayal.

An old black dog appears,
in my life, as I rush to turn pain off,
not fully realizing, this
one action robs me of the beauty,

of the light at night. I wonder, is my
home ruined
by having it built
too tight?

SHIFTING GROUND!

Life's pressures, shift us away,
from encountering those inner maps,
which Spirit beckons us
to travel.

Distractions honored, keep us
free-floating, moving
only with the most pressing
issues at hand.

Participating in shifting,
from the vital,
depreciates our sense of the
important.

An inner driven power, influences
us into the multitude of goods,
at the expense
of the best.

Straying like paper blown
from place to place,
caught in the winds
of disorder.

AN UNSAVORY FORCE

Listen! Listen!
I confess I am
captured by an
unsavory force.

Talk tells
of my burdens,
anxiety is tearing
at my heart.

Strain appears
on my brow,
struggling to make
contact meaningful.

Caught in the trap
of my role,
the sounds I hear,
are the noises of addiction.

Deafening noises,
keep me distanced
from the very
heart of God.

Dulling noises,
keep me away
from talking honestly,
about me.

Me in relationship
to the Divine,
who will help
me break addictions?

A TROUBLING PRESENCE

Boredom is full
of cutting devices:
emptiness, alienation,
loneliness.

Boredom creates
a loud cry for change,
in ourselves, and somehow
in all of what we do.

Boredom's primary root,
drives us to make promises,
keeping us objective in our quest
of the discovery of knowledge for change.

Boredom pulls us away from
feelings, feeding the need we think to
be rational.... its poison
has caused us to forget.

DUCKS: MY WIFE SAYS DON'T TALK TO STRANGERS

Seeing a Mallard, a pure white
duck with one little duckling left of the brood____
all three have taken me under
their wings since my arrival.

The adults came running up to me
today as though something was needing
to be said or was going to happen
soon.

Voices of loud quacks, quacks, convinced
I understand; they slowly turn and
walk toward the spraying fountain,
accompanied by choice, and gladly welcomed.

EMOTIONS

A human necessity, without,
not able to experience fully
alive moments with self or
others.

Emotions carry us on the
drastic rides of life, immersing
us in intense emotions of shock,
doubt or surprise.

Emotions bring us to the
deepest of connections as we
share love in another's arms,
reassured, all is ok.

Tragic, if we live life
without them, be ready
here they come with some cost
to each of us.

No way around it.
Life isn't easy, having to
watch for tacks and splinters
along the way.

FOUNTAIN

Here at St. Andrew's Abbey,
you have become a daily
companion of my spiritual
journey.

I've sat often with you,
open to entering a relationship.
Knowing, I hear your
voice in the water.

Hard work since you
don't ever move toward me.
It is always about my willingness
to move closer to you.

I've strained to listen, to
be awake, for anything you
might say. Then I hear, we are
all, droplets in the grand scheme.

All of equal importance. The choice being
ours, trembling in fear, facing the large
fall to be a "Joyful Moving Celebration of
Love."

DROPLETS

It's so pleasant in the
quiet places of the fountain.
Kept so clean and
clear.

Oops, where are we going?
Oh, down into the darkness.
But still
moving.

Incredible speed, pressure,
squeezing us,
for some unknown
task.

Where are we headed,
what will happen to us?
It's uncomfortable,
too close, then it's over.

Over the edge, flying through
the air____ laughing, wondering,
who empowered us with such
possibility?

SILENCE IS TOUGH

Silence can be deafening
as two people set across
the room, not knowing how
to respond to the clamoring noises,

bombarding each other's minds.
It distances them from the chaos of
hurt, the deep sadness, consuming
their lives.

Caught by the trap of missed
opportunities, which may have
led to greater love. Does talk
have any real hope toward healing?

Walls are thick, fear has driven
them apart. Will they give passion
permission to rise? Can they risk
fresh air, to heal their brokenness?

DEEPER SUBTLETIES

Searching has always been exciting!
Will the wonder of discovery
be found around the next corner,
under the next turn?

Significant noticing will appear
as time is given to recall all that has
been seen. Both clear
and unclear.

Excitement wanes as the journey
onward emerges; our hearts know
great discoveries are made along
lived paths of life in the ordinary.

Arrival, though exciting, pales in the
intense emotions experienced,
in the challenge of the forward
movement.

QUIET CONTEMPLATION

Stillness, is no escape.
It is an immersion into
life's fullest reality; stillness
moves toward openness.

Quiet nurtures us into
an abiding intimacy with
ourselves. Knowing self
needs love first.

Quiet moves us beyond ourselves,
into the mystery of wonder, giving
space for healing
toward action.

GRACE IN CHAOS

Havoc bred this frenetic activity
looming high over our heads,
with the price of disconnect from
God and others.

Pushing us away from
commitment, not nurturing self in Spirit,
increases
our sense of helplessness.

Overwhelmed by personal choices,
withdrawing into anger, feeling stuck
with depression gripping my life,
I turn into the dark mystery.

My heart opens to sacred space,
feeling pushed into the stillness,
discovering, an unfamiliar experience
of love and affirmation.

The gift of a
"Word" read... speaks directly
into my heart with healing and
hope of return.

DOOR

It feels massive to me,
this door ___ containing
such mystery, in its
opening.

Tension pulls at the
center, begging
to be swung open,
to its full capacity.

Encountering risk,
as I embrace
change,
openness feels overwhelming.

Remaining closed I can feel
secure, breathe normal,
experiencing the
predictable.

The grand closed door,
represents immense
possibilities, to open,
risk, to hold closed,
safe.

DESPAIR ENTERTAINED!

Poets must never
run away from despair.
My mind turns on its own
inward journey.

Despair, feeds anger,
God allows his
closest friends to be prone
to anger.

Despair pushes
into our experience
of personal
poverty.

Despair requires of us, a
humility about who we are
and what we do. Thus, life
is captured fully.

Understanding ourselves
better, giving more
freely, knowing a humility
we can stand in.

LIFE IN DARKNESS

Life is also discovered in
darkness and silence,
such able companions
on any path.

Life's energy plies us toward
trust, and silence
toward a new experience
of listening!

These moments are the
first discoveries of Grace.
Our eyes open to the beauty
of the late evening sky.

Darkness and silence, present
in all creation. Welcomed, they
are full of surprises, discovering
a renewed vision.

These, make up the door of
discovery, the Divine is our
breath, flashes of light cause
us to hush, opening our hearts.

Silence is the testing fire, tasting
delicious terror toward the darkness,
which comes to shape our heart
desire to prepare us for God's love.

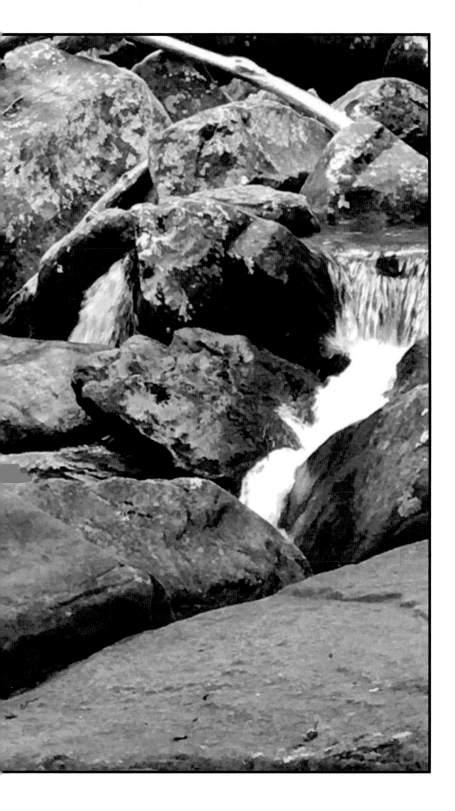

TWO

SCRATCHING LINES

Despite the medicinal poetry, there is death everywhere (in life and in my poetry.) I try to grapple with meaning – how do we find meaning when pain abounds?

SILENCE

Silence births a grander
hope, it pushes the
noise away to discover
peace.

Silence beckons us to let go
releasing what we think so
important.
For the Divine knows.

By letting go, we open
ourselves to Divine Embrace.
It reveals what distances us from
the very heart of God.

It disrobes us,
calling all of us to
celebrate the fullness
of our lives together.

SCRATCHING LINES

Scratching, is about searching
for You in the time of
silence,
away from routine.

Tossed up between
fellowship and silence.
Caught by our need for intimacy
and comradery with God.

Words flood our minds
with little of significance,
as our hearts
ache for more of
You.

Words distance us from the reality
of Your Presence.
Why choose noise rather
than the encounter of Your silence?

CALL

She said, "I want to work with
troubled women." Her call in
the moment, God's voice ringing
from the past.

Confirming direction comes,
though costly, little did
we know of the warfare, already
in the making.

Moved ____ increased problems
____ asthma, tightness ____
difficulty
breathing.

Low air, anxiety,
fear! What next Lord? Will
I be healed? Will low air be my
limit in life? No! NO! No...

ANWAR

"I am not going to make it!"
She reported, words from his
mouth, which tear like a barb caught in
the warm flesh of the afternoon.

"I am not ready to hear them," turning
them away like the
sound of branches scratching
on metal.

"My heart aches for all of us standing
by his bed," his hand touches her cheek,
"I don't think I am going to make it!"
"Too soon to go, we have much to do!"

Anwar shares:
"This is my dream, someone
is taking my tree away. I love this tree and
I am going to take it with me.

No, I love it and hope to keep it,
but the tree is gone,
my heart aches, beyond measure.
Why is prayer answered this way?"

Anwar's death leaves me feeling alone,
the emptiness cries out
from my heart with unembraceable pain.
His voice brought love.

From his dream about
the tree came love.
Love is what
took him away!

LONG APART

It has been too long
with all the stuff of life
impacting each of us.
Yes, there is a perceived strain
in being with each other.

We try old ways of being
and it doesn't seem to make any
difference. Yes, it is difficult
to be with each
other.

Wondering how to connect….
Pain overwhelms my heart,
will we ever be connected
again? Have we grown
too far apart?

What made the energy between
us?
Where has it gone?
Out of rhythm, we say.
What does it mean?

Simple movements that are
clamoring, clumsy, crude,
not smooth, reflective
of our journey
apart.

WHAT DO I DO?

Stand by bedsides,
looking into faces,
feverish, and laying
on cumulus pillows.

Called to confront ____
the demonic darkness
that jabs of sickroom
greenish light.

My heart gasps
when a contending
element chokes their
utterance.

Why does it feel like
cheating, as I
celebrate my 57th
birthday?

No, you don't
frequent my thoughts,
but deep in the nerves
of my body.

I hear a loud cry,
of too soon passing,
sallow faces, thirst for life
and I too thirst!

THE VINEYARD

I wondered as a child,
if Jesus played in the
vineyards of his home town.

Did he play hide and seek?
Did they play tag together? Jostling
about, with those he would later

choose as his disciples,
watching them hunger
for more of God,
I wonder….

RABBITS

Two, hopping into the small
space of lawn where I sit.
They are hungry, for a late
day round of green grass.

Seemingly drawing closer,
maybe to share, about
their day near the
retreat center.

Returning to my reading,
I hear a scuffle, as they are off
for the race of their lives.
Heart beating faster, coyotes are near.

Speed moves them from their near
death experience. The Creator knew speed was
necessary, for distance builds
toward safety.

It seems they move in reflection
and prayer now. Moving toward home,
telling of their adventures today.

Simply, a hole
in the ground,
joining family for a
dream-filled rest.

SMOLDERING EMBERS

We find ourselves
setting together
awaiting
the evening
meal.

There arises
the ever-present,
smoldering embers,
that keep us distanced
from each other.

Soft jazz plays
in the background,
quietly surfacing
over the human chatter,
that surrounds us.

The waitress
attempts to comfort us,
as our order, and our lives,
go through another delay.

There is an artificial sense about
all of this activity, as they set close,
making feeble attempts at community.
I notice, in the eyes of

those who walk by, the
undercurrent of
loneliness
and isolation.

Those attempts at community around
a common table, shattered
by the inner storms
of our lives.

RETREAT EXPERIENCE

Grieving over her life
experience, now …
sick… low air,
blocked … Why! Why!

Why this intensity? Why
spiritual companionship?
In a flash, given awareness,
increased burden.

Health, out to crush her call,
her life, any price, doesn't matter,
STOP! An alive woman longing
to serve broken women.

Health issues, Yes!
Medical history, Yes!
Call!! Now!!
Struggle for breath!

Intercession, protection,
overshadowed, by the
mighty protector, who
has already said, GO!
Serve!

SPIRITUAL DIRECTION

Praying for each other
everyday! A new
covenant of noticing God's
gracious work in her.

She came open, challenged.
"I am being stretched," she
spoke softly of God's active
molding influence.

We both knew.
Graced times
enriching,
nurturing.

She began to walk deeply,
graciously, lovingly;
she became
Divine changed.

FIVE MEN

Men voluntarily
choosing to step aside
from their hurried lives
and work.

Moving to the unhurried
in hopes
of discovering the Divine
anew in the quiet.

Discovering struggles
to find God in the chaos
and noise of their uncomfortable
places of existence.

God abides in places, where the
Divine woos us into hearing
the still small voice. Longing
for intimacy with us.

Encouraging us to return
to these hopeful places where
we can be together
with God.

For Sherry

GRIEF

Preoccupied, she walked into the
room, sorrow weighed heavy
on her heart, caught by the death of
her mother.

Professional, in her own
right, recognizing
her need
to journey with loss.

She entered robustly with
attentiveness, questions,
risking a fish bowl ____
everyone watching.

Wow, discovery, insight,
movement profoundly given,
as mother, from her memory
spoke release to her daughter.

CHRISTIAN FAITH

Christian faith in this
house is a joke, living lies.
People say it's important,
but live with no effective results.

Faith is
an albatross about my neck,
I want something which
works in this terrible storm.

Clarity is always elusive,
over-sought, simply wanting
something that works, better
than lies.

Abraham, Issac, Jacob, will any
of your religions work for me
In these troubled times? i am
becoming a holy thief, and this works.

DARKNESS

The veil of darkness
quickly envelopes
us. Feeling desperately
alone.

Clouds
hanging low,
almost touch
the earth.

Hearing the sound
of faint
voices, a gentle
roar of the cooler.

The evening bell tolls,
calling us to Compline
entering a grand
silence.

Let the darkness
enter, friend to friend
it asks of
us.

This repeating
exercise, causes so
many to fear
rather than rejoice.

Darkness walls us
in, left anxious
by its
presence.

Darkness in its
eternal rhythm,
longs
to enfold us.

Why, oh why
such resistance?
God
is there!

LOSS OF KINDNESS

Kindness is trickling away,
lost in the swift embrace of change,
plowed over by our sense of
insecurity.

We easily hide behind our doors,
not looking over our neighbors'
fences, cars slowly move by, as
paranoia raises its ugly head.

We embrace, as a friend, the fear of
the unknown, holding creative
exploration at a distance, suspicion
has become our password.

Conversations, seldom occur, though
often empty, meaningless exchanges.
Escape, rests at the core of our
interactions, now fearing closeness.

Taking back what has been lost requires
courage, facing the obstacles, creating
honored desires with change of self
and the community.

CHILDREN BEARING THE CROSS

Broken yesterday, pushed
off its place of
presentation. Shattered
in front of me.

Sadness grips my heart,
something treasured,
so easily
destroyed.

I saw how fragile life is,
what becomes important
to us so easily broken by my hand,
shaken, by how sudden it happened!

Holding life loosely, not
protected, vulnerable, with the
abrupt, casual
touch of another.

The image, full of mystery,
most who saw it,
didn't respond. Now it is
gone from our sight.

A HALF-ROTTEN ORANGE SPEAKS

She is dropped off,
told she had to stay.
A Spirituality, Pregnancy Retreat,
I noticed her embarrassed face.

Greeted her warmly, "I am only 16,
clearly not a place I want to be."
I invited her to simply settle in,
"find whatever works for you."

Nature and birthing caught her attention.
She begins to explore, picks up a half-rotten
orange, gazing for some surprises...
Deep connections made, causing tears to come,

"My mother sees me as the rotten half,
unclean, pregnant out of wedlock.
I have discovered a new freedom,
I am not unclean any longer, today, I feel
healed!"

"THE BIBLE HAS A WAX NOSE",
Martin Luther

Wax is pliable, twisting it to my own
liking, misrepresented by my own
imprint, confronted by my own
preferences.

Such vulnerabilities are often
unknown to the reader...
It is easy to turn the Book into
the ultimate solver of life's problems.

Often misapplied, out of context,
satisfying our own whims.
Easily getting lost, missing the
deep connections with the Divine.

The Book, given to show us the
Way, may it always have priority
over our thirst to easily satisfy
our own needs.

MOUNTAINS

They greet us every morning,
as the dawn bursts into
a new day. Stark and rugged
they are.

Ever sure, always
present, showing us
their stability over time,
through the long haul.

Who said we could remove
mountains? Where are ours
hiding, which Spirit wishes
to be removed?

Quietly placed in the shadows,
in the fury of living,
one forgets only
for a while.

Not given freedom of expression,
they occupy large spaces in our
lives, while we wonder about
the nudges toward freedom.

Entrusting the hard work of removal,
to the Spirit who knows well the territory
of our shadows, our fears struggle with
emptiness, with its lostness.

THE OUTDOORS

Wind gently blows
around my body. A
crow caws in the distance
telling us he is watching.

Subtle noises, roar in the
distant air conditioner near
the convent, also touching my ears,
with the occasional rumble of a car.

Mountains rise in the
distance, demonstrating their
stability as a vow____
never to leave this place.

Vast open fields lay
before me, longing for
the plow, calling forth, please
plant us so harvest can come!

INTIMACY

She is an elusive quality
in life. Mystery is
always near, but often
out of reach.

She longs to be close
but effort often falters,
under the protective eye
of another.

Intimacy risks being held.
We tremble with excitement,
doubt with
uncertainty.

Tears well up in us,
as we touch into this
mystery without
comprehension.

Intimacy's journey, draws
us deeply into the unknown,
with God and self. Yet, being
open to come to know Love.

NIGHT DRAWS NEAR

I am sitting in the opening
of my garage, facing west.
I see little impact of the
economic meltdown.

Life, 90 miles west of L.A.,
has little changed, but an
unhealthy confidence has risen,
"All will be ok."

Few of us move in healthy
relationships, an occasional wave
of the hand, a quick smile, little
time together.

Employers demand more with less.
Fences separate us. More tragic
are the walls, which divide us.
Our struggling with the unknown,

increases our fears, of the truth, of each other,
fear of the unstated and unheard. Fear robs us
of the ability to stay focused, which uproots us
of our groundedness, selling all, to simply exist.

LEAVES

The gentle rustling of leaves,
under the intense cold of
winter, are moments full
of change and beauty.

They explode into bright
yellows, flames of gold,
hallowed orange, showing
us the wonder of change.

Morning sun, shines on
brittle leaves, leaving behind
the cold of night, saying,
let go, let go, come and join us!

Leaves fall with a wisdom of
knowing, embraced by
grace. How is it we miss
their guidance?

Taking their last breath of air,
now lay matted, together
on winter's floor, crackling
under our feet.

They welcome their end, no
difference between oak, or aspen,
captured by their hopefulness,
this going each fall is not hard after all.

Trees have an inner peace about the
work of nature, they deeply sense
spring is always just around the corner.
making for a welcomed entry.

A ROUGH GATE

The creaking of the gate
opens my heart and somehow
settled in place, it rests
quietly.

Thick, wide and brownish,
for the first time noticing
its place at the center
of my life.

Hesitating, wondering,
what will be found, if my hand
is given toward
its full opening.

Did I leave anything behind?
Were there places of no-regret
in by-gone days?
My heart longs for rest from exploration.

My heart hopes, as the door
opens, for renewed hopes,
walking in fresh new places,
full of excitement.

Alone with Gratitude?

An impossibility. What begins
with the self, begs to be
shared with others.
Gratitude is not singular.

A missing component, at
least when it is very young,
not given time to fully
develop when it is shared.

Eyes dimmed by the rush of
life, often not noticing its
significant aspects, when gratitude
shared.

NO ONE SPEAKS INTO OUR DUST ANYMORE!

Tragic, broad, mysterious
consequences, no one, speaks
into our dust
anymore.

Dust, earth, clay,
the beginning elements of
creation, left behind our
ongoing formation, rooted in love.

Settling for tough skin,
crusty bark which assures us,
we don't need any other hands to
continue our formation!

Quiet please with the initial work,
afraid of life's necessary revisions,
the unknown feeds
our lack of pursuit.

Wondering, _____ a woodpecker
breaking through the crusty bark,
digging a deep hole, to implant
new hope in our lives. Wow, what happened!

FATHER'S TOUCH

Each of us seek after him,
as we fall from our mother's
womb, we ache
for our father's touch.

Fathers make choices to
move in love toward us or,
disappear into their own
demons, though always present.

Sought after in the distance
between decisions he makes,
caught in the wind
between whatever.

Will we know more of ourselves,
if we find him? Longing to be touched
by his hand, a look of tenderness,
entangled in the hairs of his beard.

Occasionally, he lovingly touches us,
with the warmth of his eyes, the nod of his head,
the tenderness of his hands, so seldom.
Can we endure the loudness of his rage?

BROKEN OPEN

Seeing an old photo of our
three children enjoying the
backyard pool. My heart
bursts open with intense emotions.

I have forgotten those days, as the
years have come and gone, noticing
the awe of joyful experiences
gone by.

Our lives molded by illness, surgery,
struggle and death,
shading my eyes, for a time,
struggling to see.

Knowing life's commands, keep awake,
alert, attentive, live in the
present, as I struggle to simply
take my next steps.

Hanging in, provides
an intimacy, giving new ways to
see. Gratitude is the gift
through the messy experiences of life.

THE ROOM OF LOVE

Love rooted in openness, plus
inclusivity, breaks open the
quality of its essence.
Welcoming those who wish to enter.

Walking together
provides a diversity of experience,
deepened through the doorway
of change.

Only through love, can
the ages of spirit, be encountered
with the hope of gathering
a sliver of wisdom.

Love is always
being rearranged
by those who
enter.

BIRDS

Our chirping tells others,
you have entered our space.
Watching you over many months,
some days seem light and free,

others so heavy, we fear for you to break.
Humans, a complex lot,
creator has blessed us with ease,
enjoying the brightness, of the moment.

Knowing, not to hold onto the present, for
it soon passes, living with the anticipation
of something new to appear. We have no room
for moments of fretting, our little bodies too small.

Hopefully
you sense
our gift
to you... take it, make life lighter.

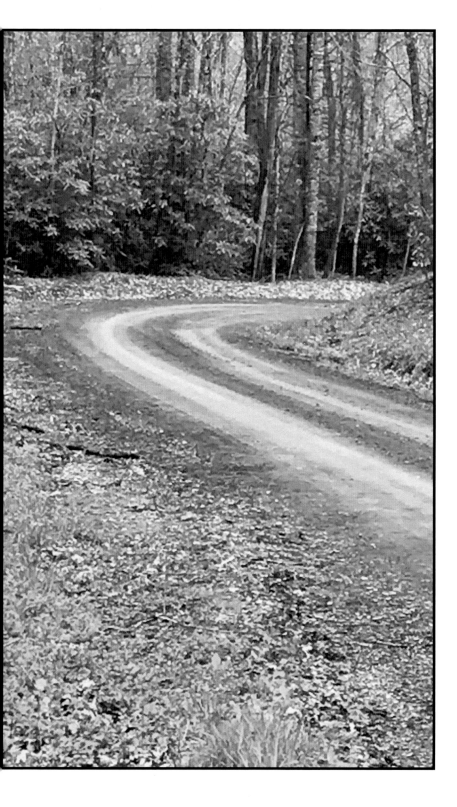

THREE

SOMETHING GREATER

This is my promise that despite this pain, there is still a bit of faith that I hold. This is the "awakening" and "acceptance."

SACRED PLACES

Sacred places
call us,
beckon us, woo
us into them.

Sacred places
are known for
marked grace
toward inner peace.

Sacred places
nurture us,
stir and challenge
us toward healing.

Sacred places
tell us to
let go,
hold life lightly, be open.

Sacred places remind us,
change that is real,
is often not
willed.

TRAGEDY! THEN NEW LIFE COMES!

September 11, 2001 the World Trade Center
attacked and destroyed. All in shock,
overwhelmed,
full of grief.

Torn by all the happenings,
September 12th,
our hearts are drawn toward
home.

Rebecca is in labor we are told,
on the whirlwind of war you come,
little Michael David,
6lbs 12 oz you are.

Letting our world know by
your cries, you are early,
you have not been made to feel
safe and secure in mother's arms.

Through pain and tears you
come reminding us. All is not
lost, all is not over. Our shock
gives way to joy, fears to trust.

Small you are, one month early
they say, you come to us
weak and vulnerable, but you
too change our world.

MUSINGS WITH FANTASY

The Stations.
Walking them,
discovering
new images.

Hopping.
Rabbits hopping,
       wonder,
floods my imagination.

Do they recall
what happened
that day?
       I wonder!

Do they long to
soften the blows, as the
earth shook in fear?
       I wonder!

When he saw you
enveloped in pain,
what did he think?
       I wonder!

What you saw
that day, you
never recovered.
       I wonder!

Leaving you anxious, fearful,
never fully
at ease!
          I wonder!

What does he think now
watching from
another place?
          I wonder!

MOTHER'S CHALLENGES

I noticed a young mother opening the
door, coming out of the house across the street.
She had in hand the newest little person
of their family.

His head touches a little above her knees,
passion rests in his actions _____ he
wants his
independence!

She carefully protects him from the near
curb, knowing the fall would
cause great pain! Her body hovers over his
as they walk together.

Using her hands and arms to assist, in
necessary balance, keeping him
on his feet. Not sensing her love at the moment,
arms flailing in the air, resisting her control.

She smiles, knowing well his intention.
As he jostles along, his face is alight with the
smiles and laughter with his
new found freedom.

SLEEPING MICHAEL

Asleep on a
blanket, on the
floor,
a baby boy.

My grandson
so still, breathing
quietly, as
a seven-month-old would.

He feels ok
to sleep,
deeply,
trusting.

Trust deepens
in all of us
for we are family
you see and he knows it.

AN ODE TO NONA

She entered my life, by the wave
of a hand, and
a smile, so
full of delight.

Hunger and hurt were
the common themes,
from many aspects of
life.

We discovered a soul connection,
hearts acknowledging a deep
trust, from which we longed
to share.

We moved into retreats, teaching
others from this place of health.
Asking the Spirit to nurture
us along the path.

Many have discovered this wonder,
of union life, deepening faith in
the mystery called God, sensing
profound wisdom and joy added to life.

KATHLEEN IS 3 NOW......

Kathleen
the little girl sitting
quietly on the floor, outside
the room where Gilbert lay.

Kathleen, is the
silent observer of
her family's grief,
over the death of this man.

Kathleen looks so
forlorn, not really
knowing what to think
or feel.

I kneel down
look into her lovely
brown eyes, introduce
myself, making contact.

Kathleen turns her eyes
away, uncomfortable with the
intensity, but turns back.
I ask her name, her eyes brighten.

Kathleen repositions
herself, watching my every
move. She somehow
knows we both need

the reassurance of this
new friendship, to
get through this
ordeal.

SUSAN AND KEN

Oh, what a surprise
comes in the night.
Oh, what joy
to see what was conceived.

To feel her body,
to sense new life.
To know this is ours,
can we believe it?

The thrill of new birth,
floods us with new emotions,
change in our lives,
closeness we feel.

Overwhelming,
wordless,
this rapture
has come to us.

This life given
is ours to share,
to nurture, influence,
to direct and care.

God, give us wisdom,
in giving ourselves, to
see her mature and
grow.

May we remember
this gift is ours
for a moment
of time.

Joyful, as she takes her
place pursuing life's
quest, grant your
Spirit to complete our
sharing with her.

LAMENT

I feel Presence, sharing
in the sorrow griping Juan's heart. "My wife died today!
Concepción represents
39 years of beauty, loving relationships,
mothering. Our pain is in seeing her last days
filled with anguish and sorrow." "Why?"

Standing at the foot of her bed, Sharon
gives a brief memorial in Spanish.
No funeral, not sufficient funds. Tearing at
their hearts knowing this last time together.

Confronted by their despair, knowing I only
sense some of their loss. Her sister-in-law,
Juana stood weeping, inconsolable,
saying her final goodbyes.

Shaken to reality, God chooses to
walk, in whatever mess life throws at us,
holding us when we do not
notice or even care; the pain is so great.

As our life experience pushes us toward the
edge, with unsure ground, feeling
overwhelmed. This is where our hope resides,
when nothing is left, but to trust.

PAIN TOGETHER

Touch into loneliness,
sensing pain, feeling
fragmented, struggling
with her.

Hooked easily by my own
brokenness, reacting rather
than acting, out of personal
failure.

Weary of the struggle as
my heart aches, too heavy
to bear, lost to those I love,
unsure of ways to connect.

"Break through my resistance,
help me discover your blessing,
through a healing word, and
see our hands together."

IMAGES

What we see,
barely visible,
interest to emerge,
to see fully.

Seeing, demands
truth, justice
beauty,
in discovery.

Seeing,
brings the
power, to
shape consciousness.

Seeing requires
honesty,
recognizing
its power.

Seeing calls, to
be intentional,
giving direction to
what shapes us.

LIFE

What is this experience we call life?
So short, fleeting and gone.

I watched a man die today,
just 28 years old. I watched him
over the last 12 months, destroyed
by the subtle killer Cancer.

He was a fighter, engulfed in the
struggle with his own spirit, to let go
and give up life. He cried this is too
early, not now, no!

He finally, captured a vision beyond
all reality, though fraught with pain
and agony, he pushed for more love,
deeper relationships, closeness.

He strove for an inner peace only
possible through love, he
discovered inner peace as he
took his last breath.

It will come to him in another time,
in another place, the finding of a new
vibrancy as he experiences, life's
mystery, beyond the grave.

MOVING TOWARD SOLUTIONS

We long to be removed
from the problems of
our lives, we desire this
most!

Often caught by
the heaviness of
conflicting energies.
Lost sight of what was happening.

What are these tests about? Who
is giving them? I am drawn toward
moments to embrace edge. I realize
it has power to overtake me.

As new eyes are given, seeing
clearly now, I discern I have
walked my way into solutions,
perceiving the importance to go with what is!

GREEN HEART _____ A GIFT.

It's from me to you,
she said,
probably from another
country.

Obviously not expensive,
those who designed it,
produced it, sadly earned
far less than you or I.

But a gift _____ anyways.
Green is an ok color for the
heart. It speaks of a soft mood,
points toward growth.

Pleasant to hold, easy to be with.
Who knows what one
might find in the
simplicity of a gift?

FRIENDSHIP

Her smile was alive and welcoming!
She came. Not knowing at the time
to touch, to help,
to heal.

Spiritual journey was born
with each other, unfolding,
in deeper respect,
care and love.

Departure was on the horizon,
a painful parting.
The depth of bonding, new
in this relationship.

Foot-washing, the closing
ritual, equals sharing in the
sacred moments of touch,
cleansing, and healing.

Holding each other, not knowing
what lay ahead.
An intense farewell___ closing
the door _____now weeping.

SOMETHING GREATER!

Mary Ann was her name,
each of us knew her well,
her kindness, failures, impatience,
smile, her life was complex but we chose to give.

A little bit of each of us has died with her.
What grips us today, forms
our conversation. We feel left alone,
empty, she is gone, died at 3 am.

Our hope, presses us on, talking about
life's unfairness. We each hope to grow.
Because of this loss, she forced us to
consider our own end.

CANCER

Cancer is elusive, unseen,
as its ugly head surfaces,
it says, "I am here to awaken
you."

The cry heard, in each of our
hearts, is a cry for life.
Whatever treatments given,
give us life.

Our history of knowing
presses down on us,
with much awareness of
others, doesn't bring peace.

Cancer calls us to let go of
the extra baggage of life,
welcomed or not,
never easy.

Attachments, must go,
if there is hope
of healing, for
energy to flow freely.

WELCOMING WHAT'S COMING

A new year challenges me,
to walk a new path,
full of mystery and
uncertainty.

Today, nothing seems clear,
but a deep felt sense of
direction, from where I
do not know.

The chilling breeze touches my skin,
fearful of the next step, this edge sharpens
the acuity of my being. The path is
unclear to my eyes, a thick fog,

rests heavily on my future. Will I
trust this inner sense of movement?
The sound of moving air, beckons me
to the edge to fly. I leap, flooded with joy!

Suddenness, is not an experience,
I seek out on my own. I know I experience
abruptness as negative, without pleasure.

Epiphany ___ a heightened experience
of meaning, rooted in surprise, with a
breath taking notice of something happening.
Slow down, let life surround me with new energy.

STILL FINDING A HOME!

Through the fog of the early morning,
our movements stir the residents of this
home as they begin their day. The tree
has died, but it still houses life.

With open eyes I am being taught again
by mother nature. Her challenge today
is not to give up hope _ it can be found
in these unlikely places.

Under close examination, it appears
the old dead tree still provides
comfort and protection from the
elements, encouraging the pursuit of life!

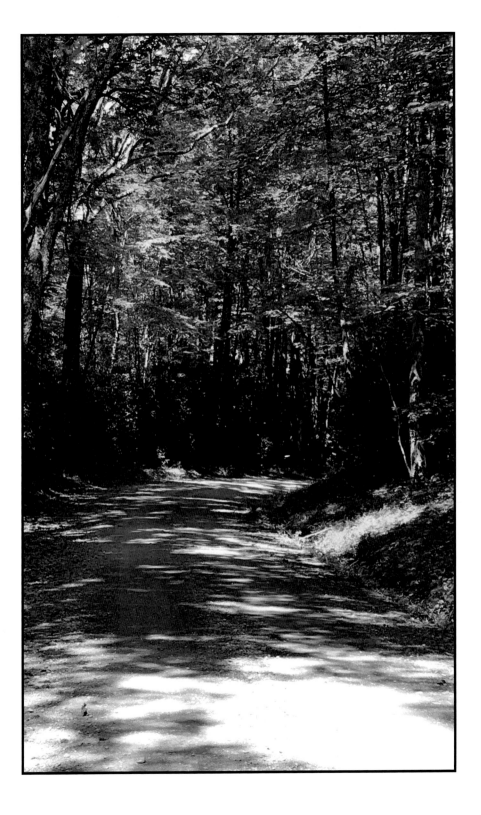

ABOUT THE AUTHOR

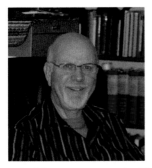 The Rev. Dr. Alden E. Sproull is from Monaca, Pa. He is an ordained Elder and pastored churches in Pa for eight years before entering Clinical Chaplaincy. He holds a B.Th, and M.Div degrees, graduate studies in Pastoral Care and Counseling at Pittsburgh Theological Seminary, and Adult Education at Roosevelt University in Chicago.

He holds a Doctorate in Christian Spirituality from San Francisco Theological Seminary, received in 2003.

His primary ministry has been with patients in hospitals and medical clinics dealing with Cancer, providing emotional, relational, and spiritual support during the journey with a life threatening illness.

Out of this ministry grew his work as a Spiritual Director. He currently has a private practice in Shelby, seeing interested persons in person and online.
He has held Prayer and Spiritual Retreats around the country.

He has lectured at the University of California Riverside in the Medical School teaching physicians Spiritual Assessment and Diagnosis, and taught at the graduate school of Psychology in Anaheim, CA. in the area of Spiritual Integration in Clinical practice for postgraduate students.

He and Victoria moved to Shelby 4 years ago to be closer to their daughter and three grandsons in Kings Mountain.

His interest in poetry began as he would hear his father read him poems written for the family to enjoy.

As he began ministry in hospital, poems began to be part of healing for himself as he found words to express what he was dealing with in others 'care. This focus was also found helpful at the bedside, assisting clients in writing their poems. Thus this book of poetry is given with the many clients in mind who helped write with him the written verses.

Made in the USA
Las Vegas, NV
27 December 2020

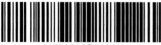